Simplified Solution Approach

To

HYPOTHYROIDISM

Empower Your Journey to Wellness: An In-depth Resource for Nourishing Your Body, Recharging Your Mind, and Embracing a Vibrant Future

Dr QUENTIN GLYN

Table Of Contents

CHAPTER ONE
Hypothyroidism

A medical disorder known as hypothyroidism is defined by an underactive thyroid gland, which results in inadequate thyroid hormone production.

The thyroid gland is a butterfly-shaped structure in the neck that secretes hormones that are essential for controlling a number of body processes. Numerous symptoms and health problems may arise from the thyroid gland's inability to generate enough thyroid hormones.

Knowing What Hypothyroidism Is:

Definition and Overview: Hypothyroidism is the result of insufficient thyroid hormone production by the thyroid gland, especially thyroxine (T4) and triiodothyronine (T3).

The body needs these hormones to function properly in terms of metabolism, energy generation, and general health. Hashimoto's thyroiditis, an autoimmune disorder in which the immune system unintentionally targets thyroid tissue, is the most frequent cause of hypothyroidism.

The gland produces thyroid hormones, which have an impact on a number of physiological functions, such as digestion, body temperature, heart rate, and metabolism. A slowing in these processes brought on by insufficient amounts of these hormones might result in a variety of symptoms as well as possible problems.

Significance Of Thyroid Function:

The hormones produced by the thyroid are essential for preserving the body's equilibrium. They control how quickly cells make energy, which has an impact on metabolism and how well organs like the heart, brain, and muscles work. Growth and development, reproductive health, and the maintenance of a healthy weight all depend on the thyroid gland functioning properly.

The pituitary gland, which generates thyroid-stimulating hormone (TSH), controls the thyroid gland itself. The thyroid gland releases thyroid hormones into the circulation in response to signals from TSH. Reduced hormone synthesis results from the thyroid gland's inadequate response to TSH in hypothyroidism.

Common Symptoms: Individuals with hypothyroidism may have a range of symptoms, varying in intensity. Typical signs and symptoms include:

1. Weariness: Even after getting a full night's sleep, people with hypothyroidism often struggle with ongoing weariness and a sluggish feeling.

2. Weight Gain: Even with a balanced diet and regular exercise, a slowed metabolism might result in unexplained weight gain.

3. Cold Sensitivity: Because hypothyroidism impairs the body's capacity to regulate its temperature, it may lead to a sensitivity to cold temperatures.

4. Dry Skin and Hair: Brittle hair and dry, flaky skin may be caused by low thyroid hormone levels.

5. Muscular Weakness and Joint Pain: Muscle weakness and joint pain may result from reduced metabolism, which also affects muscular strength.

6. Despair and Mood Swings: Thyroid hormones affect how the brain functions and a lack of them may lead to mood disorders such as irritability and despair.

7. Menstrual Cycle Disorders: Amenorrhea, or the lack of menstruation, may result from

hypothyroidism's impact on the menstrual cycle, which can cause irregular periods.

8. Memory and Concentration Problems: Thyroid hormones are involved in cognitive function, and a lack of them may lead to memory loss and trouble focusing.

It is essential to comprehend these signs in order to diagnose and treat them early. For those with hypothyroidism to avoid problems and live better overall, it is imperative that the illness be diagnosed and treated promptly.

CHAPTER TWO
Reasons Behind Hypothyroidism

1. Genetic Elements:

Explanation: The development of hypothyroidism is mostly influenced by genetic predisposition. Thyroid diseases run in families, making an individual more vulnerable.

Simplified Solution Approach: Early diagnosis might be aided by routine thyroid monitoring for those with a family history. Changes in lifestyle and careful monitoring of thyroid function may result from knowledge of hereditary risk factors.

2. Immune System Disorders:

Justification: Hashimoto's thyroiditis, also named for autoimmune thyroiditis, is the most frequent cause of hypothyroidism. Thyroid function is decreased and inflammation results from the immune system attacking the thyroid gland inadvertently in this situation.

Simplified Solution Approach: Immune system control is necessary for the management of autoimmune hypothyroidism. Minimizing environmental triggers, eating a diet high in nutrients, and managing stress may all help prevent or lessen autoimmune responses.

3. Inadequate Dietary Resources:

Explanation: Hypothyroidism may result from inadequate consumption of essential nutrients such as iodine and selenium. While selenium is necessary for the conversion and activation of thyroid hormones, iodine is required for their synthesis.

Simplified Solution Approach: It's critical to maintain a diet that is well-balanced and high in iodine-rich foods (dairy, shellfish, and iodized salt) and selenium-rich foods (sunflower seeds, Brazil nuts). Supplemental nutrients may be advised if there are deficits.

4. Environmental Elements:

Reason: Toxins from the environment, such as pollution and substances that alter hormones, might affect thyroid function. Hormone synthesis and control may be interfered with when some chemicals are exposed to excessive levels.

Simplified Solution Approach: It's important to have a healthy lifestyle that reduces exposure to pollutants in the environment. This entails selecting organic meals, utilizing natural cleaning products, and being mindful of any environmental dangers.

Simplified Approach To Hypothyroidism In General:

Frequent Observation:

Plan for routine thyroid function testing, particularly in the presence of recognized risk factors or a family history.

A well-rounded diet

Eat a diet high in minerals, such as foods high in zinc, iodine, and selenium, among other nutrients that are vital for thyroid function.

Handling Stress:

Learn stress-reduction strategies since stress may make autoimmune diseases worse. This might include yoga, meditation, mindfulness, or other forms of relaxation.

Awareness of the Environment:

Keep your exposure to the environment in mind. Select organic food, make use of natural cleaning supplies, and limit your exposure to anything that can interfere with your thyroid.

Medical Advice:

Seek the counsel of a medical expert for tailored guidance and care. A doctor may recommend medication, such as thyroid hormone replacement treatment, depending on the patient's specific requirements.

Recall that the reduced solution strategy combines lifestyle adjustments with ongoing observation and, if required, medical intervention. Always seek the advice of a medical expert for specific diagnosis and treatment.

CHAPTER THREE
Diagnosis And Hypothyroidism Testing

1. Typical Diagnostic Examinations:

• TFTs, or thyroid function tests:

• TSH (thyroid stimulating hormone): Because the thyroid gland is not making enough hormones, elevated TSH levels often indicate hypothyroidism. The main indicator of thyroid function is TSH.

• Free T4 (thyroxine): This gauges the bloodstream's concentration of active thyroid hormone. Low values might be a sign of hypothyroidism.

• Triiodothyronine (free T3): Although less often measured, low free T3 levels may aid in the diagnosis of hypothyroidism.

• Antibody tests for thyroid:

• Antibodies against thyroid peroxidase (TPOAb) and thyroglobulin (TgAb): High levels are indicative of autoimmune thyroiditis, which is the most frequent cause of hypothyroidism (Hashimoto's thyroiditis).

• T4 Total and T3 Total:

• The total quantity of T4 and T3, including both free and bound forms, in the blood is measured by these procedures.

• T3 in reverse (rT3):

• Elevated levels might indicate thyroid malfunction brought on by stress or non-thyroidal illnesses.

2. How To Interpret Tests Of Thyroid Function:

• TSH Different

• Primary hypothyroidism is often indicated by high TSH and low free T4.

• In some instances, free T4 and T3 levels are low while TSH is within normal limits, suggesting central (or secondary) hypothyroidism.

• Assays for antibodies:

• TgAb and TPOAb positivity point to autoimmune thyroiditis.

• Total T3 and T4:

• When free T4 and T3 levels are unclear, these tests may be able to offer further details.

3. The Significance Of Thorough Testing

• Personal Variability:

• Individual differences in thyroid function mean that symptoms and test findings don't always match up. A thorough panel aids in evaluating the general health of the thyroid.

• Determining the Subclinical Hypothyroid:

• Some people may have mild symptoms or normal TSH levels but high antibody levels. Extensive testing facilitates the identification of subclinical instances.

• Treatment Monitoring:

• To ensure ideal hormone levels throughout therapy and to alter drug doses, regular testing is essential.

4. Getting Expert Assistance:

Specialists in endocrinology and general practice:

Personalized treatment regimens and proper diagnosis depend on consultation with healthcare specialists.

• Interaction with Healthcare Professionals:

• Give a detailed description of any symptoms, such as weight gain, weariness, cold sensitivity, and any history of thyroid problems in the family.

Monitoring and Follow-up:

• Follow-up consultations on a regular basis are crucial for tracking development, modifying medication, and resolving any issues or symptom changes.

• Dietary and lifestyle advice:

• In addition to medical care, healthcare providers may provide advice on dietary modifications, stress management, and lifestyle adjustments.

Finally, a combination of thyroid function tests, antibody tests, and a careful evaluation of symptoms provide a complete approach to the diagnosis and testing of hypothyroidism. Those with hypothyroidism who seek medical assistance, especially from endocrinologists and general practitioners, are guaranteed a precise diagnosis and customized treatment regimens. Effective treatment and enhanced quality of life for individuals with hypothyroidism are facilitated by consistent monitoring and transparent communication with healthcare professionals.

CHAPTER FOUR

Modifications To Lifestyle To Manage Hypothyroidism

A complete strategy is necessary to manage hypothyroidism, which includes modifying lifestyle choices to promote general well-being. This is a comprehensive summary of the main ideas on lifestyle modifications for hypothyroidism management:

1. Nutrition And Diet:

Diet: It's important to choose a nutrient-rich, well-balanced diet. Make sure that a variety of fruits, vegetables, whole grains, lean meats, and healthy fats are included in your meals. This supplies vital nutrients and aids in keeping blood sugar levels steady.

Steer clear of goitrogens: These foods have the potential to disrupt thyroid function. Among these are cruciferous foods, such as Brussels sprouts, cabbage, and broccoli. Though they don't have to be fully removed, you may want to boil them to lessen their goitrogenic potential.

Consumption of Iodine: Iodine is an essential part of thyroid hormones. Make sure your iodine consumption is sufficient but not excessive since too much or too little of it might have negative effects. Add foods high in iodine, such as dairy, seafood, and seaweed.

Eat Less Processed Meals: Additives and preservatives found in processed meals might affect thyroid function. Choose whole, unprocessed foods to promote general well-being.

2. Foods Good For The Thyroid:

Foods High in Selenium: The thyroid hormone conversion process requires selenium. Include foods high in selenium in your diet, such as seafood, sunflower seeds, and Brazil nuts.

Sources of Tyrosine: Tyrosine is an amino acid required for the synthesis of thyroid hormones. Lean meats, dairy, and legumes are foods high in tyrosine.

3. Supplements For Nutrition:

Vitamin D: A healthy thyroid is linked to adequate vitamin D levels. If your levels are low, think about taking supplements or consuming foods high in vitamin D, such as eggs, fatty fish, and fortified dairy products.

Because of their well-known anti-inflammatory qualities, omega-3 fatty acids may be able to lessen inflammation brought on by thyroid conditions. Consume foods high in omega-3 fatty acids, flaxseeds, and walnuts, or think about taking supplements.

B vitamins: The thyroid is influenced by B vitamins, especially B12 and B6. Make sure your diet includes items like meat, chicken, fish, and leafy greens to ensure you get enough of these nutrients.

4. Physical Activity And Exercise:

Frequent Exercise: Take part in a moderate-to-intense exercise on a frequent basis. This may enhance mood, increase metabolism, and promote general well-being. Strength training and cardiovascular activity are both advantageous.

Yoga: Including yoga in your regimen might help you become more flexible and manage your stress. There are particular yoga positions that are advised for thyroid health.

5. Techniques For Stress Management:

Meditation and mindfulness: Prolonged stress may have a deleterious effect on thyroid function. Stress management techniques include deep breathing exercises and mindfulness meditation.

adequate Sleep: Make sure you receive adequate restorative sleep. Insufficient sleep has been linked to hormone imbalances and stress, which may impact thyroid function.

Time management: Plan out your everyday tasks to cut down on needless stress. Set priorities for your work and make time for rest.

Never forget that you should always get medical advice before making big changes to your diet, exercise schedule, or supplement regimen, particularly if you are on medication or have a pre-existing medical condition. Since everyone reacts differently to lifestyle modifications, tailored counseling is essential for successful hypothyroidism treatment.

CHAPTER FIVE

Options For Medication And Treatment

Let's explore a more straightforward approach to treating hypothyroidism, emphasizing medication and treatment choices. This will include a summary of thyroid drugs, their side effects, important factors to consider, and alternative treatments.

An Overview Of Drugs For The Thyroid:

1. Levothyroxine (T4):

• The most prescribed drug for hypothyroidism is levothyroxine.

• It is a synthetic version of thyroxine, the thyroid hormone (T4).

• It aids in restoring the body's natural levels of thyroid hormone.

• Usually taken orally, ideally first thing in the morning.

2. Liothyronine (T3):

Another thyroid hormone drug that contains triiodothyronine (T3) is lithiothyronine.

• In contrast to levothyroxine, it acts more quickly but lasts for a shorter amount of time.

• For more accurate control, often used in conjunction with levothyroxine.

3. Desiccated Thyroid Natural (NDT):

• Originated from pig or cow thyroid glands.

• Has a T4 and T3 mix that is comparable to thyroid hormones in humans.

• Some people like NDT because of its more comprehensive makeup.

Consequences And Side Effects:

1. Modifications in Dosage:

• Determining the proper dose is essential and can need frequent blood tests.

• While under medication can not lessen symptoms, overmedication might cause hyperthyroidism.

2. Interaction with Additional Drugs:

• Some drugs and supplements may prevent the body from absorbing thyroid hormones.

• Let medical professionals know about all of the drugs you use.

3. Observation during pregnancy:

• During pregnancy, thyroid hormone levels are very important.

It could be essential to modify the dosage in order to guarantee a safe pregnancy.

4. Possible Adverse Reactions:

• Mood fluctuations, weight changes, and sleeplessness are common adverse effects.

• Although they are uncommon, severe side effects might include allergic reactions and chest discomfort.

Alternative Medical Interventions:

1. Supplementing with Iodine:

• Although iodine is necessary for thyroid function, too much of it may be hazardous.

It is essential to speak with a healthcare professional before thinking about taking iodine supplements.

2. Changes in Diet and Lifestyle:

• Eating a diet rich in nutrients and well-balanced is essential.

• In some people, certain foods, such as cruciferous vegetables, may have an impact on thyroid function.

3. Handling Stress:

• Thyroid function may be impacted by prolonged stress.

• Activities like yoga, meditation, and getting enough sleep may improve general well-being.

4. Supplements with Herbs:

• Certain herbs, such as guggul and ashwagandha, are thought to help thyroid function.

On the other hand, there is little scientific proof of their effectiveness, thus prudence is suggested.

Simplifying treatment for hypothyroidism entails balancing prescription dosages, altering lifestyles as needed, and investigating complementary treatments under a doctor's supervision.

To properly manage hypothyroidism, regular monitoring and open contact with your healthcare team are essential. When exploring alternative treatments or making major modifications to your treatment plan, always get advice from a healthcare expert.

CHAPTER SIX

Integrative Methodologies

Integrative methods for treating hypothyroidism take a broad, integrative view, integrating complementary and alternative therapies with traditional medical care. While seeking specific counsel from a healthcare practitioner is essential, using mind-body practices, herbal medicines, and holistic healing approaches may improve general health and supplement conventional hypothyroidism therapies.

Methods Of Holistic Healing:

Diet and Nutrition:

Stress the importance of eating a balanced diet full of vital minerals including zinc, iodine, selenium, and omega-3 fatty acids.

Incorporate foods like fatty fish, seaweed, almonds, and seeds that promote thyroid function.

As some people with hypothyroidism may be sensitive to processed foods, gluten, and dairy, thinks about reducing or avoiding them.

Movement and Exercise:

Frequent exercise may enhance energy levels and metabolism.

To enhance general health, include a variety of aerobic, strength, and flexibility workouts.

Handling Stress:

Thyroid function may be impacted by ongoing stress. Include stress-relieving exercises like yoga, tai chi, meditation, and deep breathing.

Sufficient sleep has a good impact on thyroid function and is essential for general health.

Detoxification:

Encourage the body's natural detoxification processes with antioxidant-rich foods, sauna sessions, and enough water.

Herbal Treatments:

Ashwagandha

Ashwagandha is well known for its adaptogenic qualities, which may boost thyroid function and aid the body in adjusting to stress.

Bladderwrack:

Has high iodine content, which is necessary for the synthesis of thyroid hormone.

Guggul:

May aid in enhancing metabolism and stimulating thyroid function.

Lemon Balm:

Lemon balm, well-known for its relaxing qualities, may help with stress and anxiety management.

Bugleweed:

Used historically to control thyroid activity.

It's vital to remember that herbal treatments may have contraindications or interfere with other prescriptions, so speaking with a healthcare professional before using them regularly is essential.

Mind-Body Methodologies:

Practice meditation:

Stress may be lessened and calmness can be fostered with the use of mindfulness meditation.

Biofeedback:

This method may aid in stress management by giving people knowledge of and control over their physiological processes.

The use of hypnosis

Hypnotherapy may assist some people in managing their stress and enhance their general well-being.

Therapy Based On Cognitive Behavior (CBT):

Cognitive behavioral therapy (CBT) is a useful tool for treating negative thinking patterns and hypothyroidism-related stress.

Integrative methods acknowledge the connection between mental, emotional, and physical well-being.

Even though these techniques could be helpful, it's important to collaborate closely with a medical expert to make sure that any integrative strategy fits your unique health requirements and doesn't conflict with therapies or prescription drugs.

Thyroid function must be regularly monitored in order to evaluate the efficacy of any integrative strategy.

CHAPTER SEVEN

Handling Hypothyroidism In Particular Groups

An underactive thyroid gland causes a shortage of thyroid hormones in the body, which is the hallmark of hypothyroidism. varied groups need varied approaches to the treatment of hypothyroidism, taking into account variables including age, gender, and physiological state. This talk will focus on the unique issues that need to be taken into account for three distinct groups: pregnant women with hypothyroidism, children and teenagers with hypothyroidism, and elderly people.

Hypothyroidism During Gestation:

1. Physiological Modifications:

• Because pregnancy increases the need for hormones, thyroid function is significantly altered throughout pregnancy.

• There is an increase in thyroid hormone synthesis and hypertrophy of the thyroid gland.

2. Assessment and Determination:

• During pregnancy, routine monitoring for thyroid dysfunction is crucial, particularly in high-risk populations.

Thyroid-stimulating hormone (TSH) and free thyroxine (FT4) values are necessary for the diagnosis.

3. Treatment-Related Considerations:

The recommended course of therapy is levothyroxine (T4), which aims to keep TSH levels within predetermined parameters for each trimester.

• To change medicine doses as necessary, regular monitoring is essential.

4. Risk Reduction:

• Untreated hypothyroidism during pregnancy may have negative effects, such as delayed delivery and problems with development.

• For the best possible treatment, endocrinologists and obstetricians must work together.

Hypothyroid Children And Adolescents:

1. Birth Defective Hypothyroidism:

• Prenatal screening is essential for identifying congenital hypothyroidism in its early stages.

• Levothyroxine treatment must be started right away in order to support normal growth and development.

2. Monitoring and Screening for Pediatrics:

• Throughout childhood, periodic screening for hypothyroidism is required.

- Tracking development, puberty, and mental abilities are essential elements.

3. Support for Education:

• Education on the need for frequent follow-ups and medication adherence is necessary for families and schools.

Children who get support services may find it easier to manage the psychological effects of a chronic illness.

4. Transition from Childhood to Adulthood:

• For ongoing treatment, a seamless transfer of care from pediatric to adult endocrinology services is essential.

Considering The Elderly:

1. Frequency and Mode of Presentation:

• Older persons are more likely to have hypothyroidism, which often manifests as unusual symptoms.

• There is a chance that symptoms may be misdiagnosed as age-related problems, thus vigilance is required.

2. Relations with Polypharmacy:

• Because older persons often take many drugs, there is a higher chance of drug interactions.

• It's crucial to evaluate medications on a regular basis to prevent interactions that might impair thyroid function.

3. Both Comorbidities and Frailty:

• Care should be given to the patient's general health, taking comorbidities and fragility into account.

Adjustments to the levothyroxine dose may be necessary depending on the patient's condition.

4. Frequent Observation:

• Due to the possibility of altered prescription needs, older patients need to have their thyroid function closely monitored.

Periodic evaluations have to include a thorough analysis of symptoms and a physical assessment.

In summary, managing hypothyroidism in specific communities necessitates a customized strategy that takes into account the distinct physiological and clinical characteristics of each group. For people in these particular demographics, collaborative treatment including endocrinologists, obstetricians, pediatricians, and geriatric experts is crucial to ensuring the best possible results. Encouraging awareness, education, and regular monitoring are essential for managing hypothyroidism well throughout life.

CHAPTER EIGHT

How To Avoid Hypothyroidism

It's crucial to remember that treating hypothyroidism calls for a multifaceted strategy that includes medication, dietary adjustments, and routine monitoring.

A healthcare professional's consultation is essential for receiving individualized guidance and care. This is a condensed method of regulating weight growth, cardiovascular health, and bone health in order to minimize issues related to hypothyroidism:

Controlling Weight Gain:

1. A well-rounded diet

• Pay attention to eating a diet that is well-balanced and rich in a variety of fruits, vegetables, whole grains, and lean meats.

• Keep an eye on your calorie intake to avoid gaining too much weight since hypothyroidism might slow down your metabolism.

2. Control of Portion:

• Pay attention to portion proportions to prevent overindulging. Smaller, more frequent meals spaced out throughout the day may support energy maintenance and blood sugar stabilization.

3. Drinking plenty of water

• Drink enough water to maintain a healthy metabolism and help regulate hunger.

4. Frequent Workout:

• Exercise on a regular basis to increase metabolism and help control weight.

• To improve general health, include a variety of aerobic workouts (such as swimming and walking) with strength training.

5. Compliance with Thyroid Medication:

• Optimize thyroid hormone levels by taking prescribed thyroid drugs on a regular basis. This may help with weight control.

Heart Health:

1. Frequent Exercise for the Heart:

• Include aerobic workouts in your regimen to promote heart health.

• Based on your health situation, discuss an appropriate exercise program with your healthcare physician.

2. Monitoring of Blood Pressure:

• Keep an eye on your blood pressure often since hypothyroidism may exacerbate hypertension.

• Manage your blood pressure with your healthcare team by making lifestyle modifications and, if required, using medication.

3. Controlling Cholesterol:

• Monitor your cholesterol levels and, in collaboration with your physician, control them with food, exercise, and, if necessary, medication.

4. Good Fats:

• Limit trans and saturated fats and choose heart-healthy fats like those in almonds, avocados, and olive oil.

Bone Well-Being:

1. Intake of Calcium and Vitamin D:

• Make sure you're getting enough calcium and vitamin D, which are vital for strong bones.

• Include fortified foods, dairy products, and leafy greens in your diet; alternatively, follow your doctor's advice and take supplements.

2. Exercise Using Weights:

• To increase bone density, take part in weight-bearing activities like strength training, dancing, or walking.

3. Frequent Assessment of Bone Density:

• Talk to your healthcare physician about the need for routine bone density testing based on your age and risk factors.

4. Thyroid Hormone Adjustment:

• Use medicine consistently to improve general metabolic function, which indirectly affects bone health, and to maintain normal thyroid hormone levels.

To summarize, the prevention of hypothyroidism consequences requires a multimodal strategy that includes a balanced diet, consistent exercise, adherence to medication, and routine medical check-ups. For efficient treatment and the avoidance of difficulties, individualized care plans that are created in collaboration with medical specialists are crucial.

CHAPTER NINE

Building Your Own Power

In the context of hypothyroidism, empowering oneself entails actively managing your health, being aware of your situation, and looking for outside assistance as needed.

Creating a solid support system, making use of internet forums and resources, and participating in patient advocacy programs are all essential components of this empowerment. Let's examine each of these elements in more detail:

Creating A Network Of Support:

1. Healthcare Practitioners:

Form a connection with a medical professional who specializes in thyroid issues and is both informed and kind.

Maintain open lines of communication with your medical team by discussing your symptoms, worries, and experiences with treatment.

2. Friends and Family:

Inform the people in your immediate circle about hypothyroidism and the difficulties you could encounter.

Ask friends and family for emotional support; they may provide understanding and motivation.

3. Support Teams:

Join online or local support groups dedicated to hypothyroidism.

Take part in conversations in groups, impart your experiences, and pick up tips from others dealing with comparable issues.

4. Counselors or therapists:

To deal with the emotional implications of treating a chronic ailment, think about getting professional therapy.

A therapist may provide coping mechanisms for hypothyroidism-related stress and anxiety.

Internet-Based Communities And Resources:

1. Websites for Education:

Look through reliable sources that provide current, factual information on hypothyroidism.

The National Institute of Diabetes and Digestive and Kidney Diseases (NIDDK), the Mayo Clinic, and the American Thyroid Association (ATA) are a few examples.

2. Discussion boards and online forums:

Participate in online communities for hypothyroidism on Reddit, HealthUnlocked, or Thyroid UK.

Make a connection with others who have gone through similar things, and ask for guidance on symptom management and available treatments.

3. Social Media Communities:

Join social media groups on Facebook or Instagram that are dedicated to hypothyroidism.

Adopt trustworthy reports that provide advice, insights, and first-hand descriptions of life with hypothyroidism.

4. Webinars and Podcasts:

Attend webinars or listen to podcasts with thyroid health specialists to stay informed.

Find more about the most recent findings, available treatments, and lifestyle choices for treating hypothyroidism.

Advocacy For Patients:

1. Advocacy Groups:

Participate in thyroid health advocacy groups like the Thyroid Cancer Survivors' Association or Thyroid Federation International.

These groups often provide materials, arrange gatherings, and promote greater understanding and treatment.

2. Take Part in Studies:

Think about taking part in hypothyroidism research studies or clinical trials.

Research contributions have the potential to enhance scientific understanding and result in better therapies.

3. Increase Knowledge:

Tell your own tale to help spread the word about hypothyroidism.

Speak out on social media and in your community for more empathy and understanding.

Individuals diagnosed with hypothyroidism can take charge of their own treatment, improve their quality of life, and advance knowledge about thyroid disorders by actively creating a support system, using internet resources, and participating in patient advocacy.

Conclusion

In summary, treating hypothyroidism with a simple solution method requires a comprehensive comprehension of the illness, its causes, and possible lifestyle changes. Through the implementation of a holistic approach that blends medication and lifestyle modifications, people may successfully control hypothyroidism and enhance their general quality of life.

Three key pillars are highlighted by the previously described simple solution approach: pharmaceutical management, dietary alterations, and lifestyle improvements. Thyroid hormone levels are regulated by levothyroxine, a typical medicine for hypothyroidism. To choose the appropriate dose and conduct routine progress checks, it is crucial to collaborate closely with medical specialists.

Dietary changes are essential in addition to medicine. Thyroid function may be favorably impacted by emphasizing nutrient-dense diets, including iodine-rich alternatives, and being aware of possible dietary deficits. Eating a balanced diet helps to manage the symptoms of hypothyroidism in addition to supporting general health.

Moreover, alterations in lifestyle have a major role in the management of hypothyroidism. Frequent exercise increases energy and metabolism, which lessens weariness that is often linked to the illness.

The negative effects of stress on thyroid function may be lessened by practicing stress-reduction strategies including mindfulness and relaxation. Getting enough sleep is also essential for thyroid function and general wellness.

It's crucial to remember that these pharmacological and lifestyle modifications should be made gradually to give the body time to acclimate and to provide a long-term treatment strategy that is sustainable.

Summary Of The Main Points:

Medication Management: One frequent drug used to control thyroid hormones is levothyroxine. Maintaining regular contact with medical specialists is essential for figuring out the right dose and tracking development.

Dietary Modifications: Give priority to a diet high in nutrients, such as foods high in iodine. Be aware of any nutritional shortages and think about seeking individualized advice from a nutritionist.

Changes to Your Lifestyle: Exercise often to increase your metabolism and vitality. Include stress-reduction strategies and give enough sleep a high priority for your general health.

Implement modifications gradually to give the body time to adjust and to guarantee long-term sustainability in the treatment of hypothyroidism.

Motivation And Encouragement:

Although managing hypothyroidism might be difficult, it's critical to have an optimistic outlook on the process. No matter how little, acknowledge the progress that has been made and recognize your accomplishments along the road. Embrace a network of friends, family, and medical professionals who are sympathetic to your situation and will support you in your endeavors.

Keep in mind that treating hypothyroidism is a dynamic process and that changes can be required in the future. Remain patient with yourself and recognize that every person's path is unique. Overall well-being and symptom management may significantly improve with little, persistent efforts.

Making educated judgments is facilitated by actively engaging in your healthcare journey, seeking out information, and maintaining awareness of your condition. Check-ups with medical specialists on a regular basis guarantee that your treatment plan is still appropriate and meets your changing requirements.

In conclusion, people may successfully treat hypothyroidism and have satisfying lives by combining medication, dietary changes, and lifestyle alterations with an optimistic and resilient mentality. Accept the trip, remain dedicated to your health, and never lose sight of the fact that you are capable of overcoming obstacles and thriving in spite of your illness.

THE END

www.ingramcontent.com/pod-product-compliance
Lightning Source LLC
Chambersburg PA
CBHW050744260726
48661CB00001B/407